An Ocean of Orange

By Emma Rose Sparrow

Publish Date: February 13, 2015

Editor-in-Chief: Connor Chagnon
Sterling Elle Publishing
Bradford, Massachusetts
ISBN-10: 1517510007
ISBN-13: 978-1517510008

AN OCEAN OF ORANGE

An Emma Rose Sparrow Book

AN OCEAN OF ORANGE is a collection of amazing photos - with accompanying text - that have one thing in common: the color orange!

You may be surprised how much orange exists in the world. From sweeping orange sand dunes in Africa to the beautiful Orange-bellied Flowerpecker bird, this book brings the color orange to life.

If you are an adult bookworm who enjoys exquisite photos, this book is for you!

It is hoped that you find this book worthy of adding to your collection.

Enjoy your read!

EMMA ROSE SPARROW

OTHER BOOKS IN THIS SERIES BY EMMA ROSE SPARROW

A Bevy of Blue

A Year's Worth of Yellow

A Gathering of Green

A Parcel of Purple

A Reservoir of Red

A World of White

A Potpourri of Pink

EMMA ROSE SPARROW

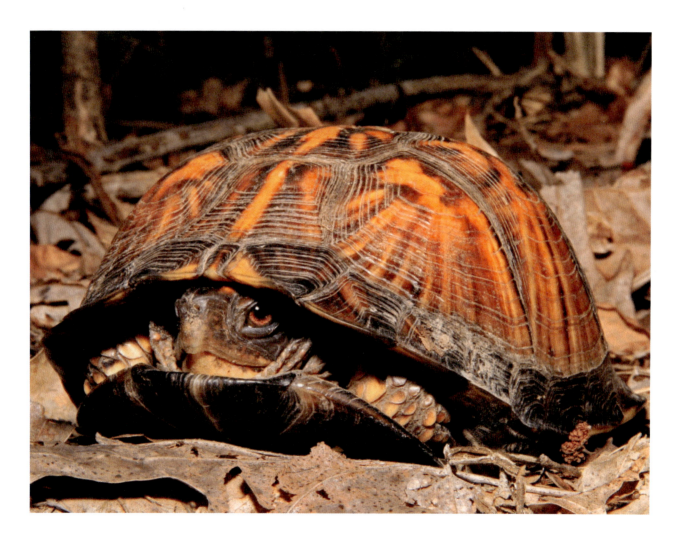

This tortoise with a shiny orange shell can be found in the Amazon jungle.

EMMA ROSE SPARROW

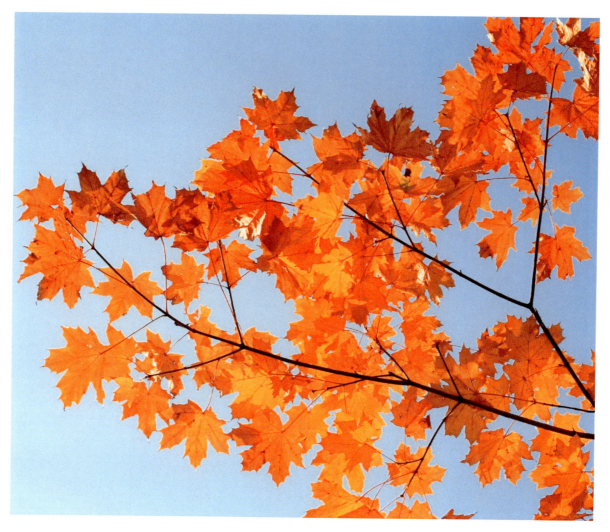

A branch of a maple tree in autumn, displaying splendid orange leaves.

EMMA ROSE SPARROW

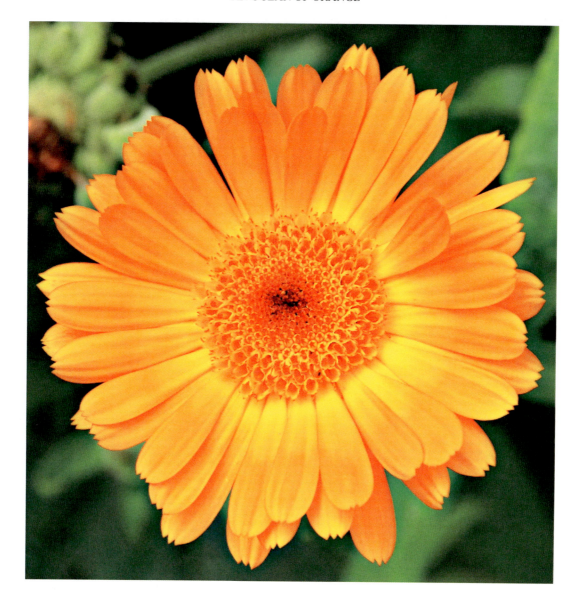

A beautiful orange Marigold flower.
In the 12th century, it was believed that just looking at a Marigold would improve eyesight and liven one's mood.

EMMA ROSE SPARROW

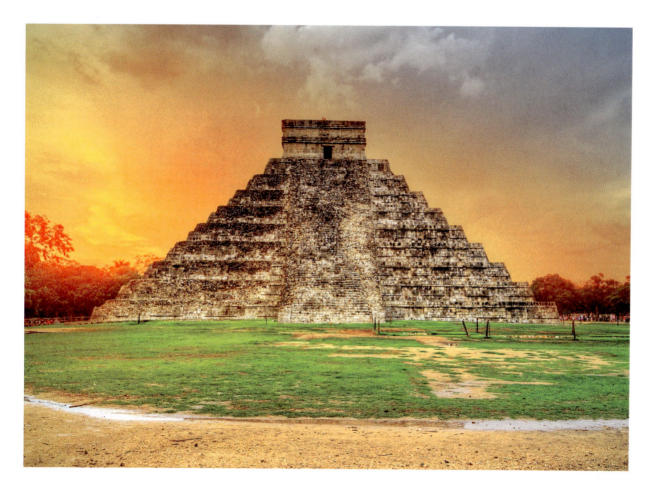

An orange sunset lends even more beauty to this pyramid in Mexico.

EMMA ROSE SPARROW

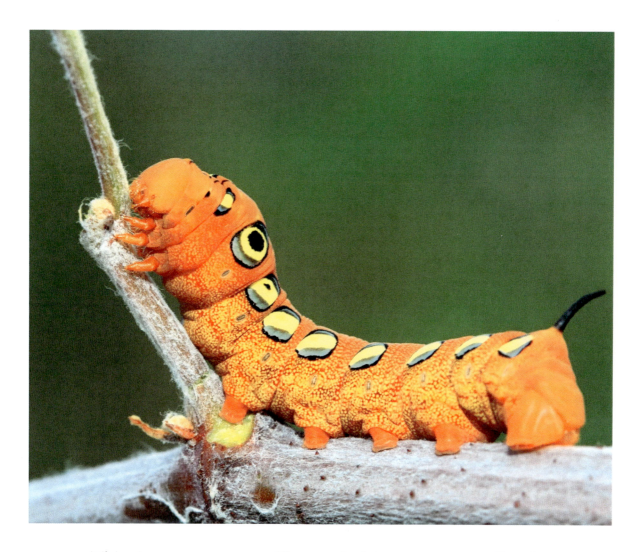

This tiny orange caterpillar works his way up a small twig.

EMMA ROSE SPARROW

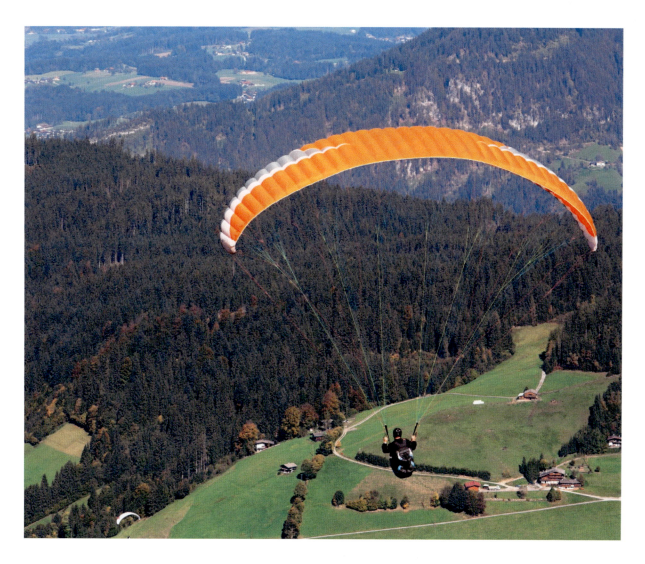

An adventurer with an orange paraglider soars over the Austrian landscape.

EMMA ROSE SPARROW

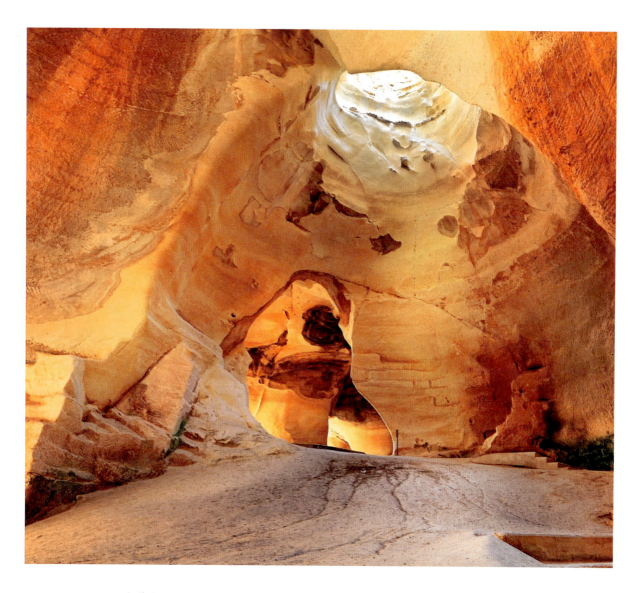

This orange rock is at the entrance of Bell Cave.
Bell Cave is located in a historical national park in Israel.

EMMA ROSE SPARROW

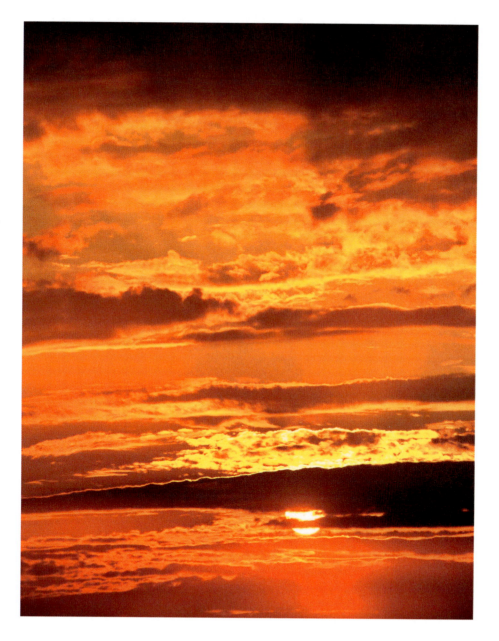

This slow sinking sun is energized with orange.

EMMA ROSE SPARROW

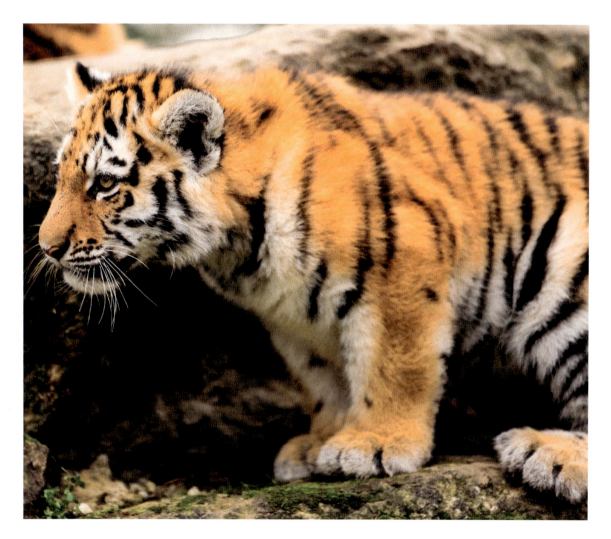

This tiger cub, with soft orange fur, is a Sumatran tiger.
Sumatran tigers are the smallest of all tigers.

EMMA ROSE SPARROW

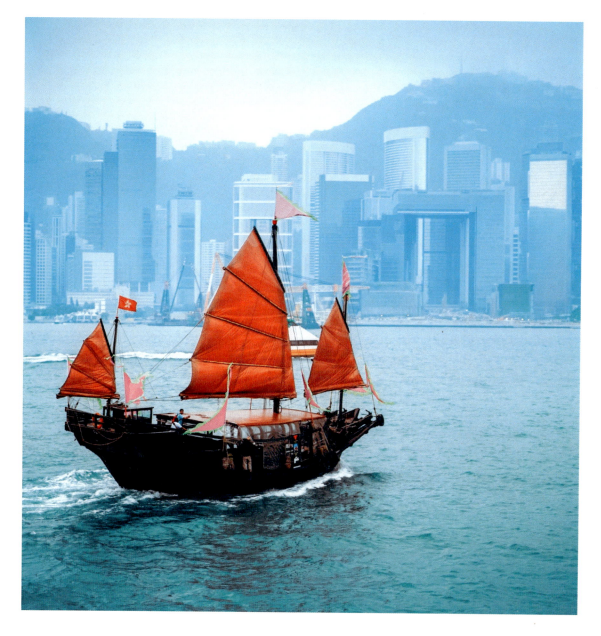

In Hong Kong, a wooden sailboat with lively orange sails steers into harbor.

EMMA ROSE SPARROW

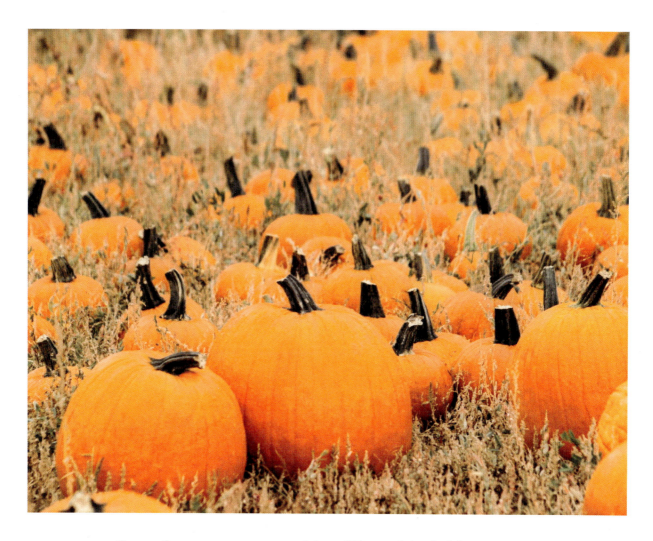

Countless orange pumpkins fill up this field in Maine.

EMMA ROSE SPARROW

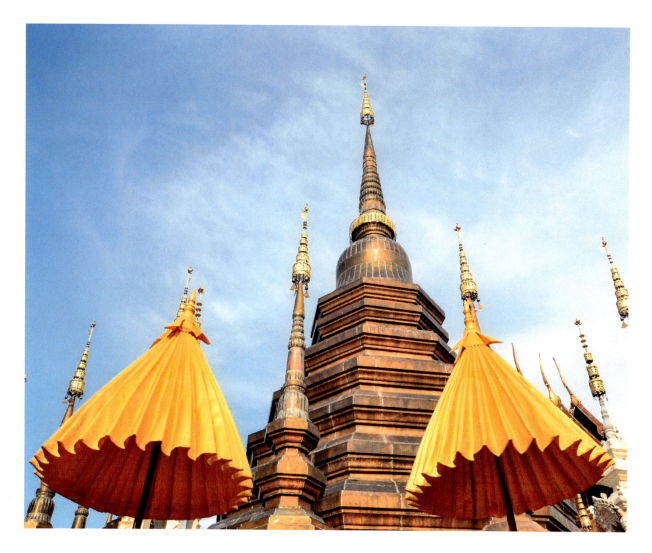

An ancient building in Japan with ornamental orange umbrellas.

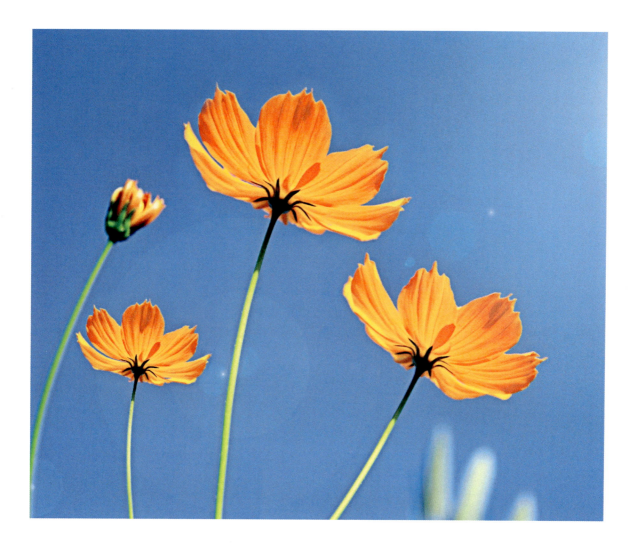

Delicate orange cosmos flowers reach up to a clear blue sky.

EMMA ROSE SPARROW

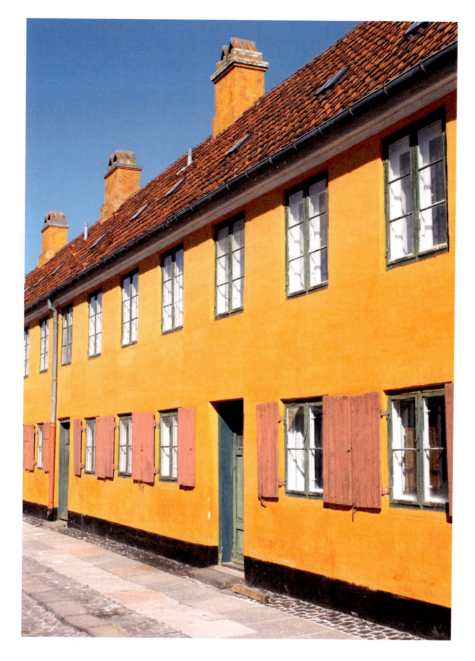

Restored orange rowhouses stand on a former navy base in Denmark.

EMMA ROSE SPARROW

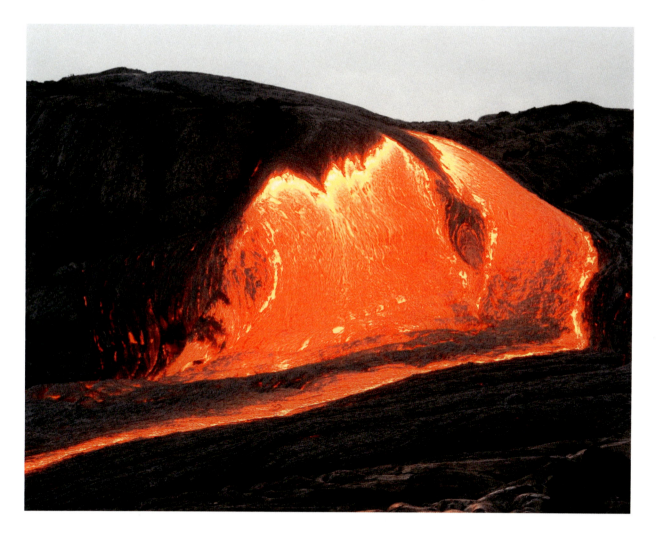

Glowing orange lava is bravely photographed in Hawaii.

EMMA ROSE SPARROW

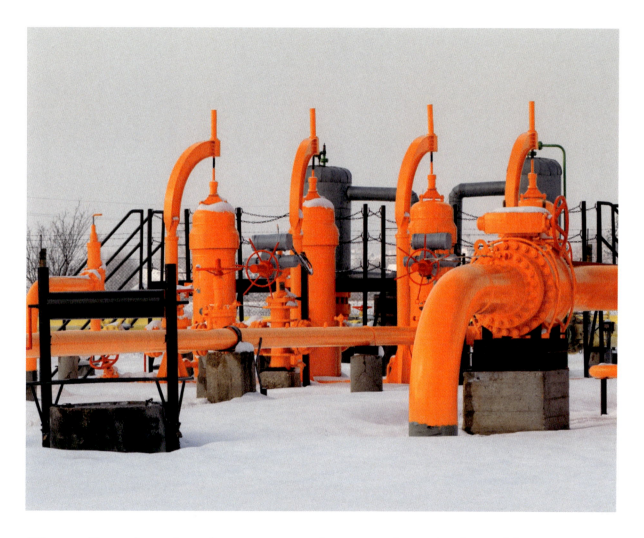

These vibrantly painted orange gas pipes stand out in the cold crisp snow.

EMMA ROSE SPARROW

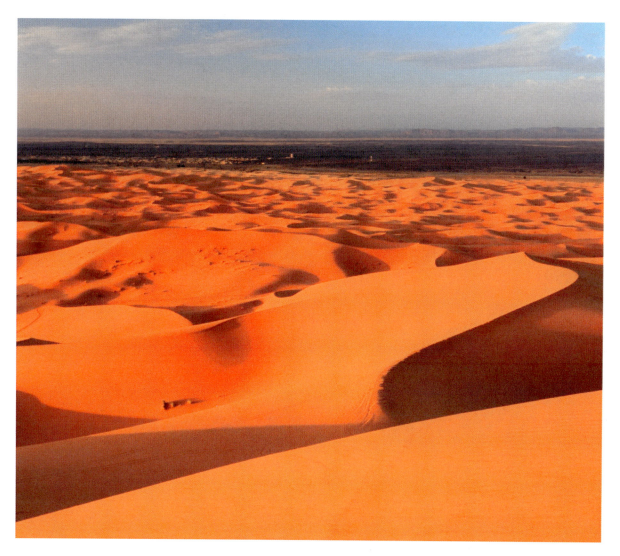

These windblown orange sand dunes are part of the Sahara desert.
The Sahara desert is the largest hot desert in the world.

EMMA ROSE SPARROW

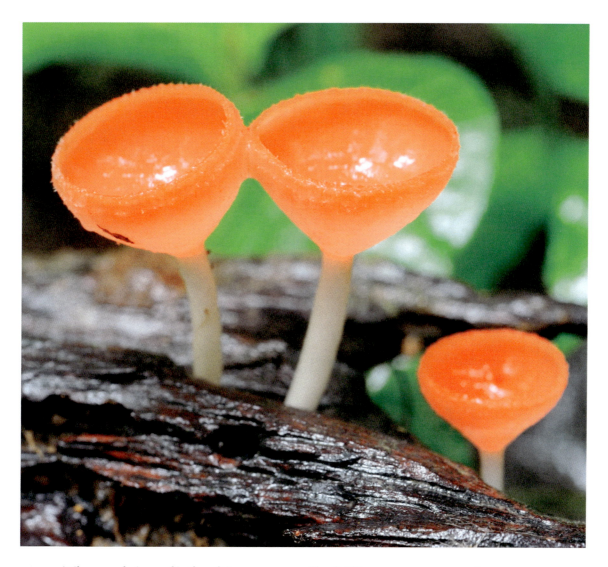

These dainty little things are called Champagne mushrooms.
Looking at the tiny orange caps,
they do look like they would hold a bit of drink!

EMMA ROSE SPARROW

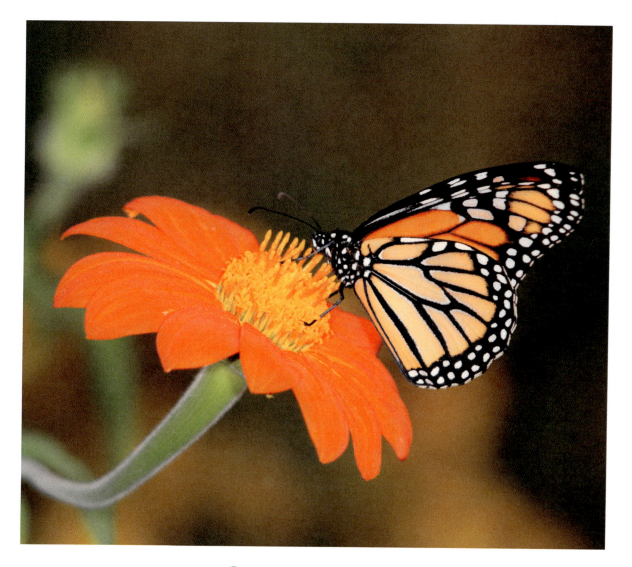

Orange meets orange!
This orange monarch butterfly seems to be drawn to his own coloring.

EMMA ROSE SPARROW

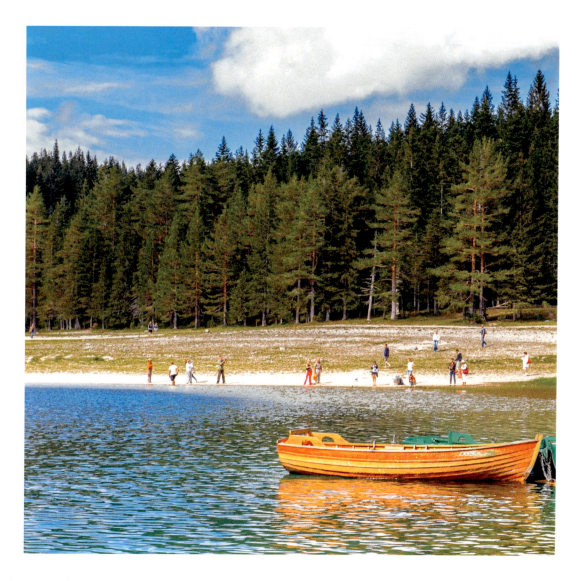

Visitors flock to the shores of a mountain glacier lake in northern Europe.
An orange boat awaits those who want to venture out.

EMMA ROSE SPARROW

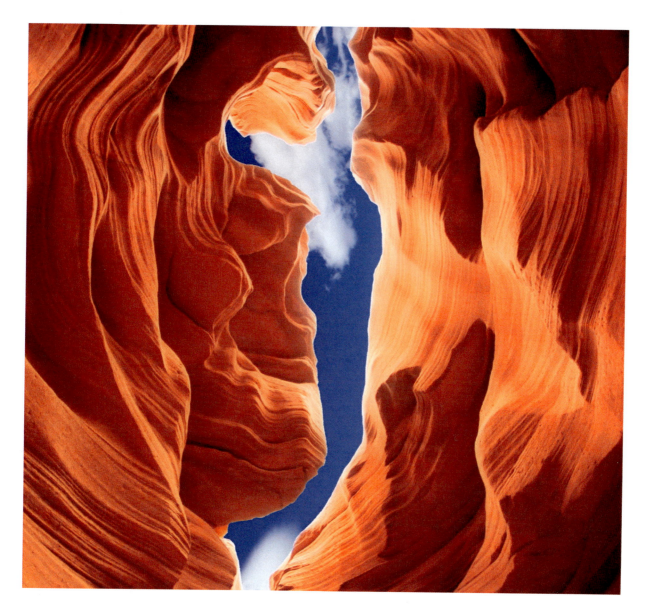

A photo taken while looking up between the orange rock walls of Antelope Canyon, Arizona.

EMMA ROSE SPARROW

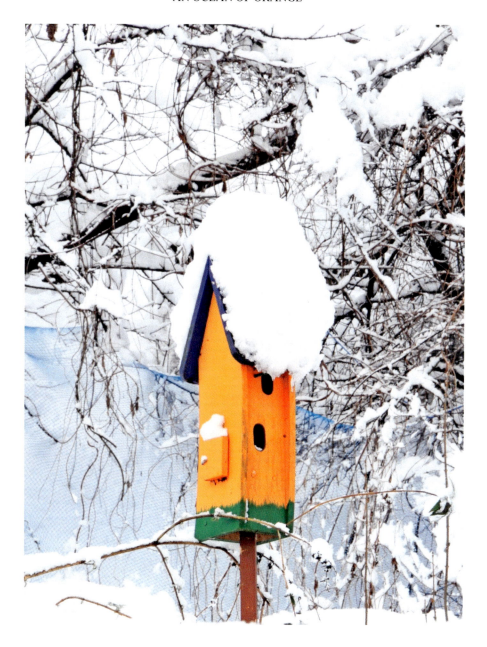

An orange birdhouse set on a post is swathed in fresh snow.

EMMA ROSE SPARROW

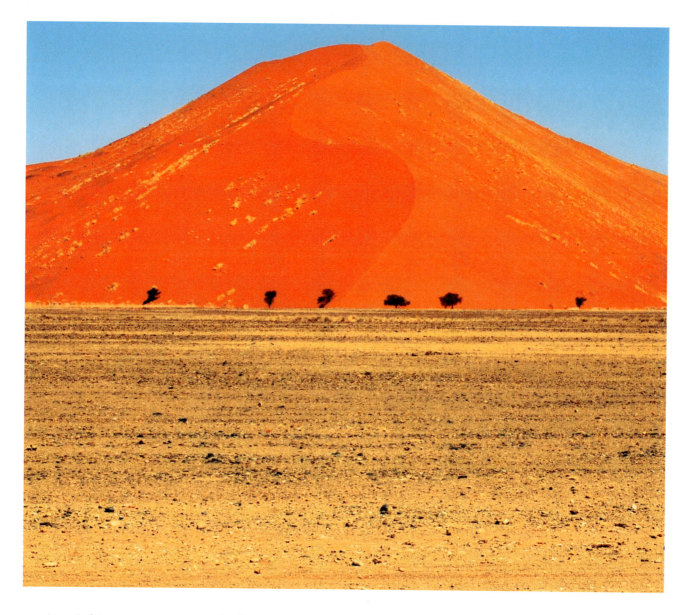

In Africa, strong winds have swept orange sand up into a towering dune.

EMMA ROSE SPARROW

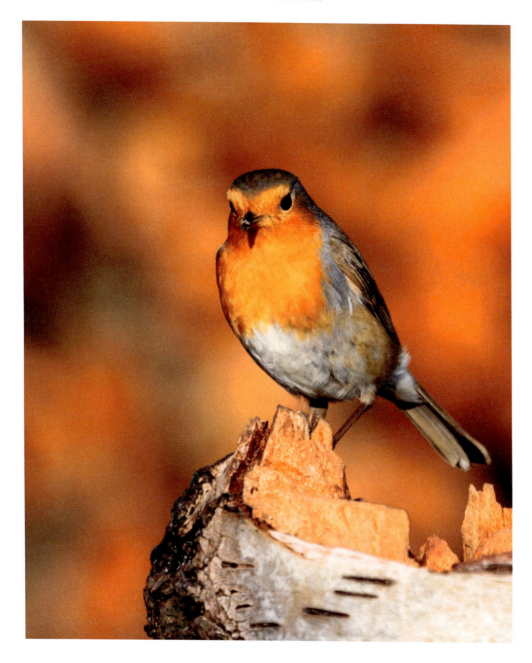

The European Robin bird has a lovely orange breast, throat and face.

EMMA ROSE SPARROW

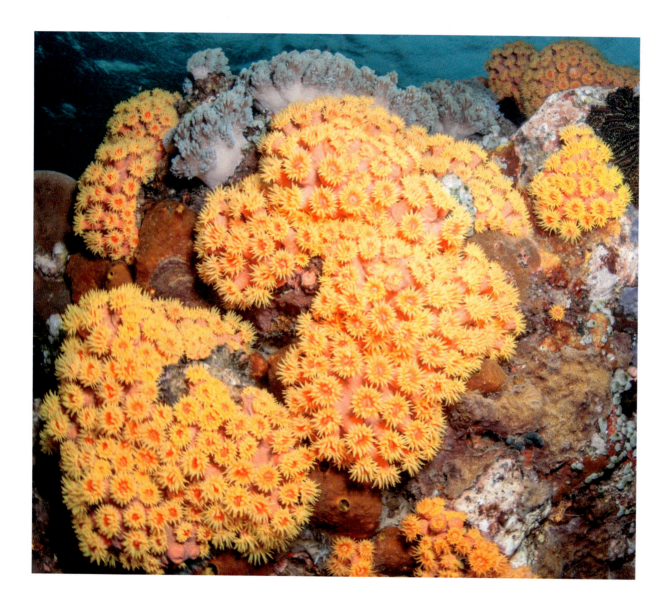

This delightful natural structure is Orange Cup coral.

EMMA ROSE SPARROW

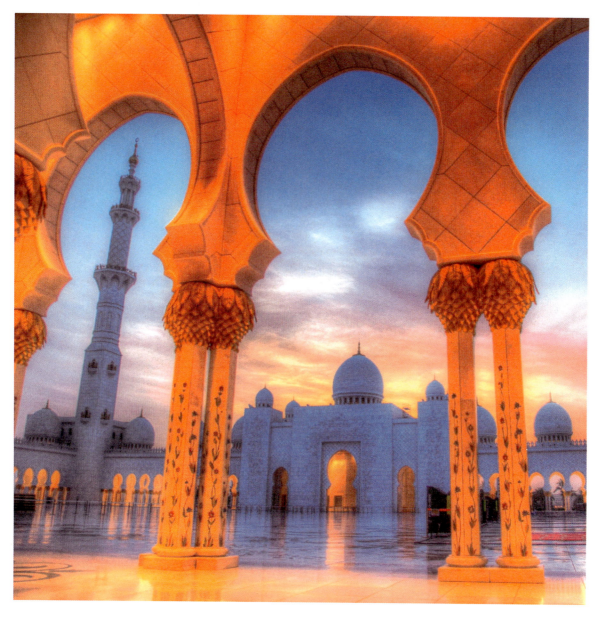

These colossal orange pillars are part of a mosque in the United Arab Emirates.

EMMA ROSE SPARROW

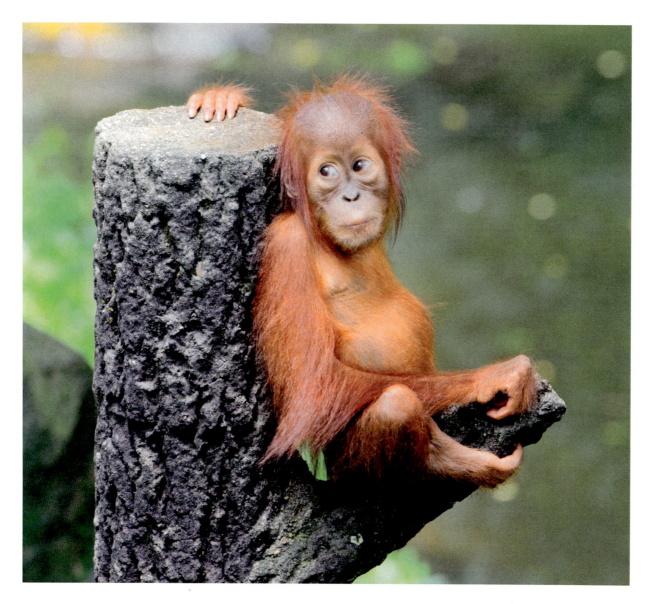

A lovable orange baby orangutan sits on a tree stump.

EMMA ROSE SPARROW

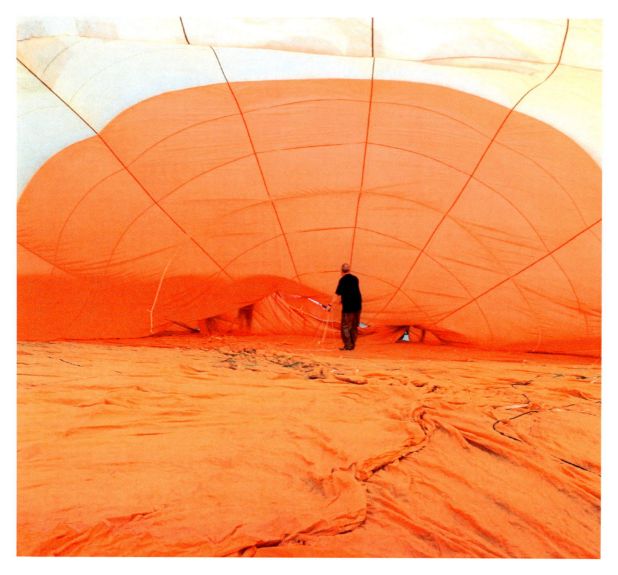

A man makes adjustments on the inside of a huge orange hot air balloon.

EMMA ROSE SPARROW

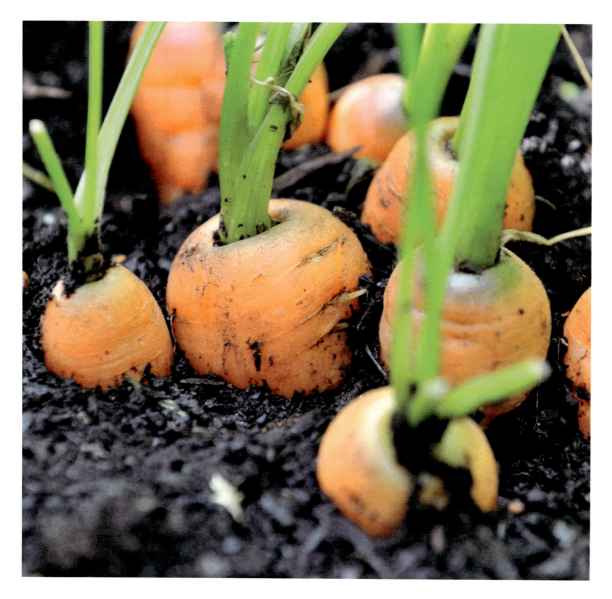

A vegetable gardener's delight!
Fresh grown orange carrots, ready to be harvested.

EMMA ROSE SPARROW

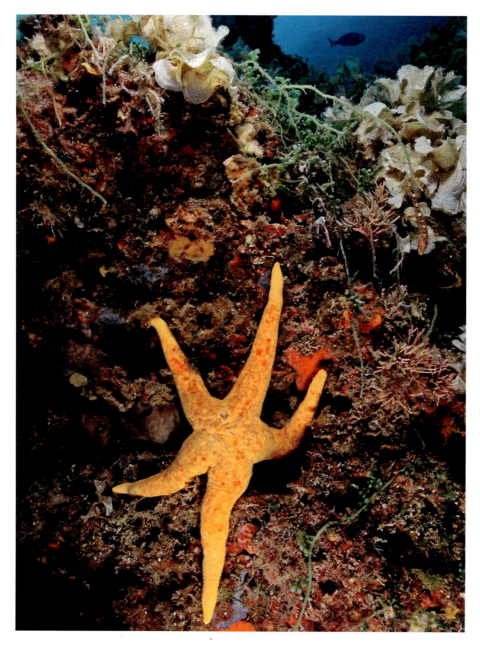

This pale orange starfish clings to rocky coral in the Mediterranean Sea.

EMMA ROSE SPARROW

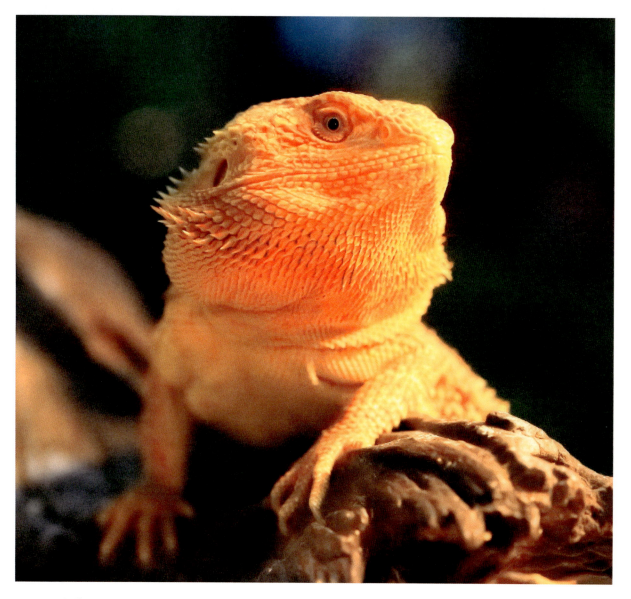

This orange Bearded Dragon lizard appears cool and collected.

EMMA ROSE SPARROW

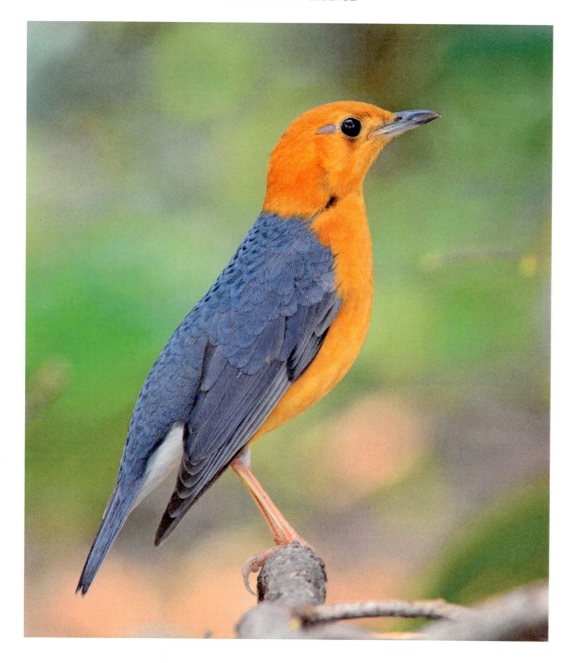

This attractive orange and gray bird is the Orange-headed Thrush.

EMMA ROSE SPARROW

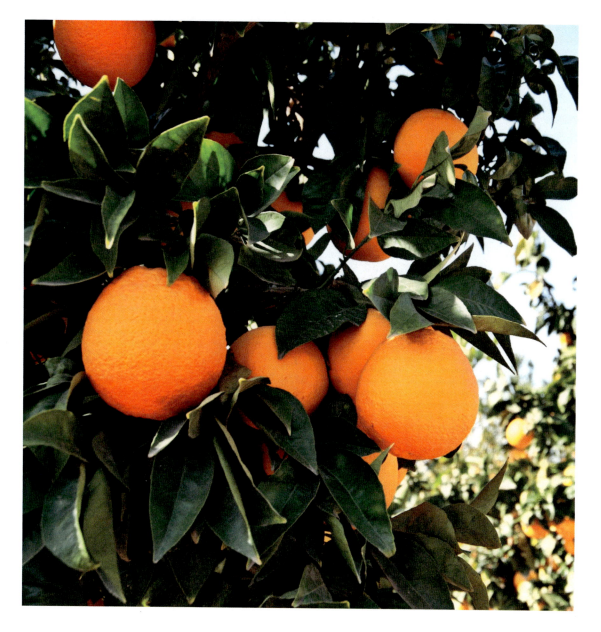

Orange trees are the most cultivated fruit tree in the world.

EMMA ROSE SPARROW

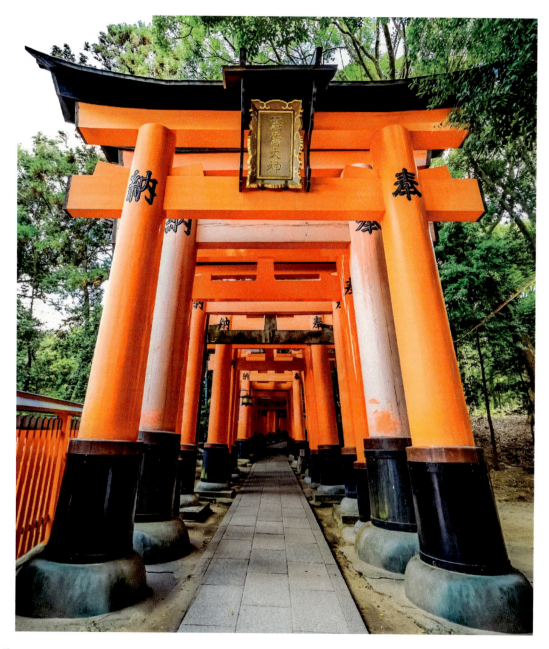

These impressive orange pillars mark the entrance to a shrine in Japan.

EMMA ROSE SPARROW

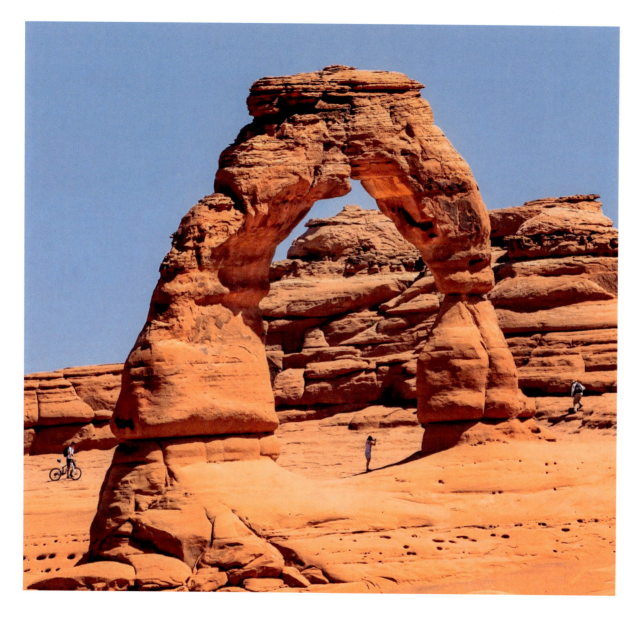

Visitors flock to this amazing natural archway of pale orange rock in Utah.

EMMA ROSE SPARROW

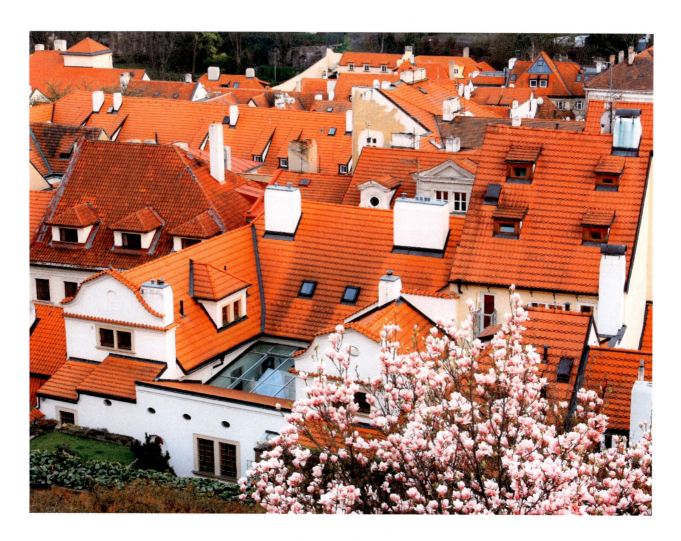

In Prague, homes traditionally have orange-red roofs.

EMMA ROSE SPARROW

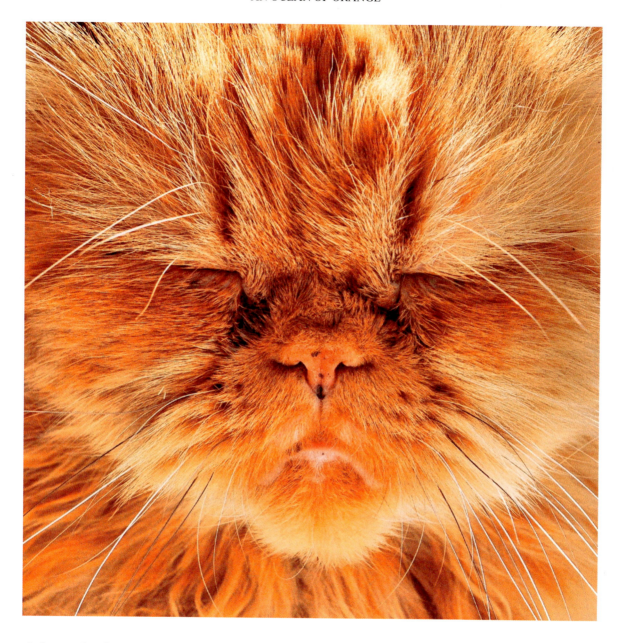

Though this orange Persian cat may be camera shy, he is just precious.

EMMA ROSE SPARROW

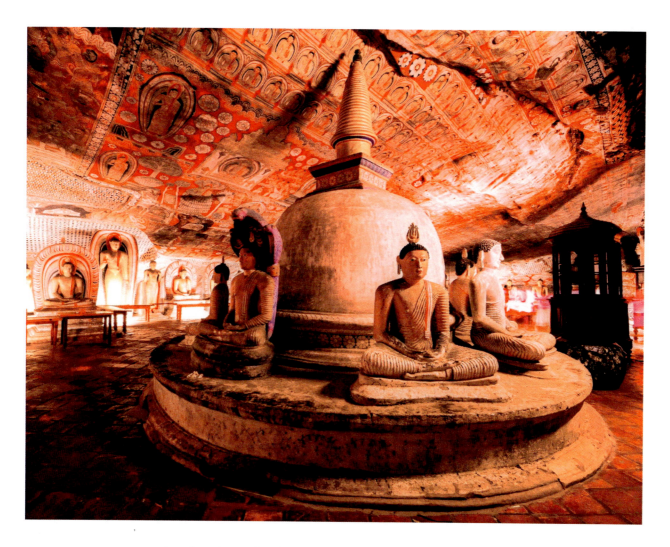

At the Dambulla Cave Temple in Sri Lanka,
there is a soft orange glow surrounding these Buddha statues.

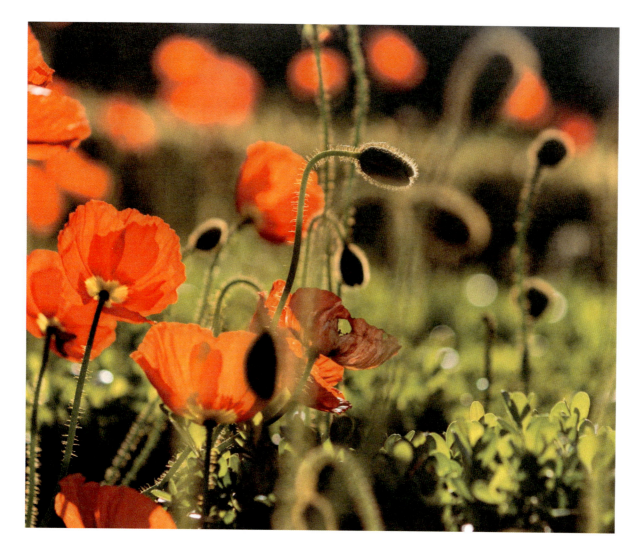

Orange poppy flowers in a meadow on a sunny summer morning.

EMMA ROSE SPARROW

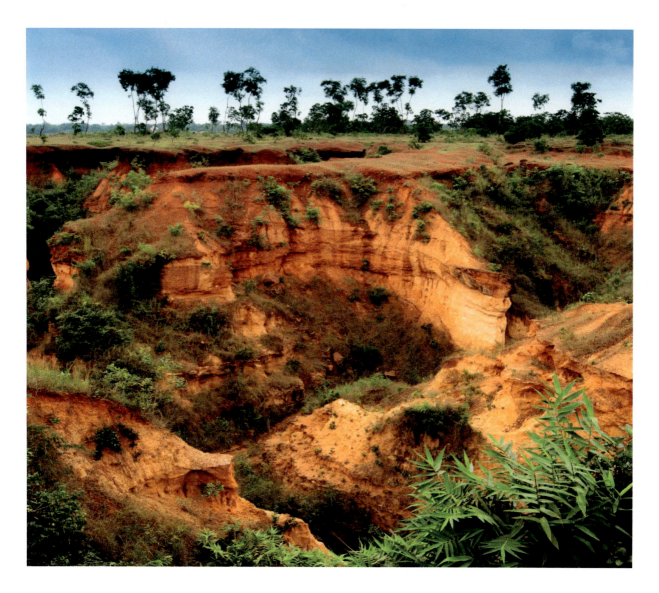

This wondrous canyon of muted orange rock is located in India.

EMMA ROSE SPARROW

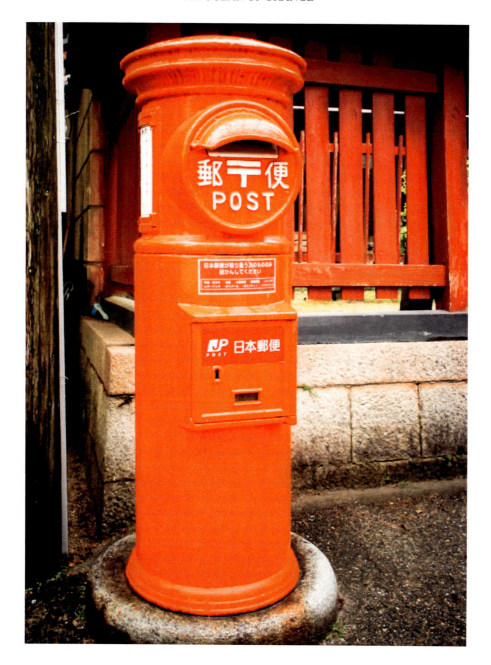

This gleaming orange mailbox is in a small Japanese village.

EMMA ROSE SPARROW

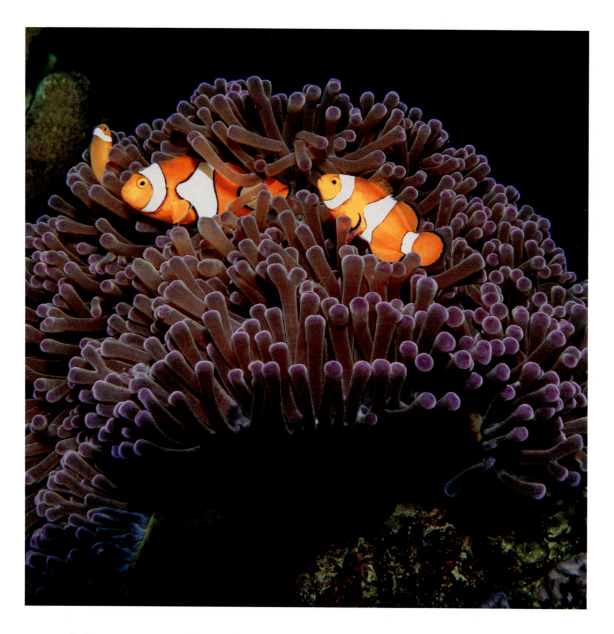

Three orange and white fish swim within soft purple coral.

EMMA ROSE SPARROW

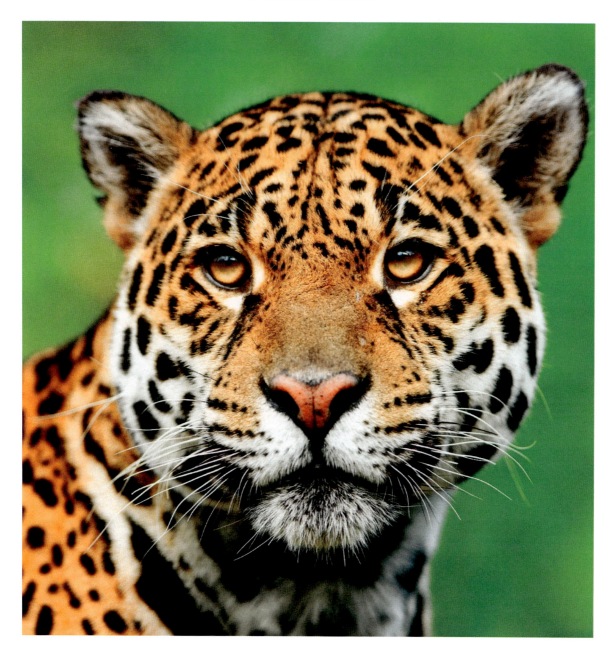

An adult orange Jaguar with perfectly matching orange eyes.

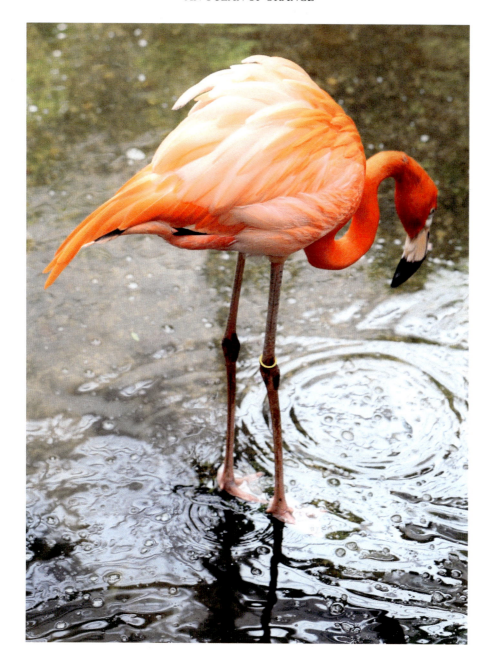

A pretty pink and orange Flamingo in the Florida Keys.

EMMA ROSE SPARROW

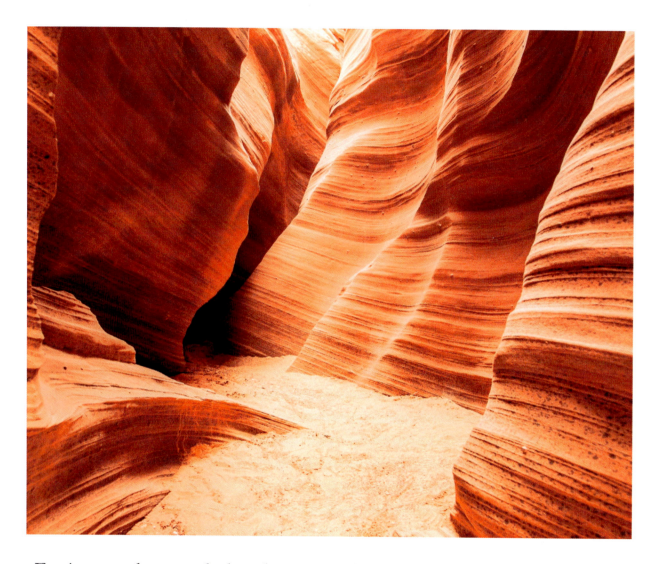

For just one hour each day, the sun sends a beam of light into the narrow, orange crevices of Corkscrew Canyon in Arizona.

EMMA ROSE SPARROW

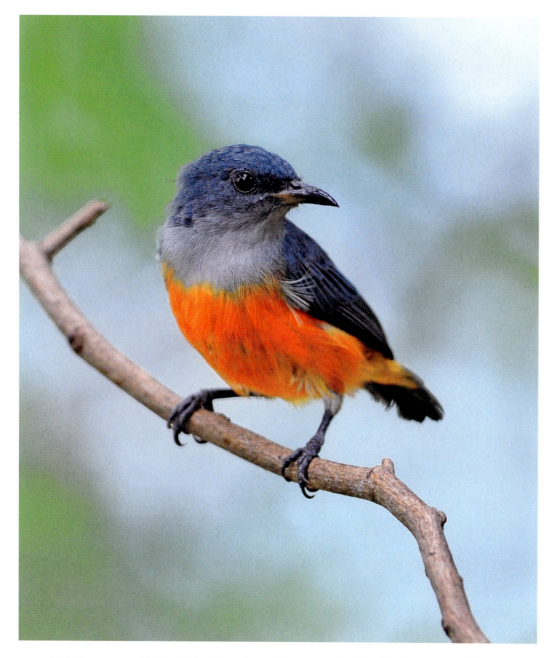

This sweet little bird is the Orange-bellied Flowerpecker.

EMMA ROSE SPARROW

OTHER BOOKS IN THIS SERIES BY EMMA ROSE SPARROW

A Bevy of Blue

A Year's Worth of Yellow

A Gathering of Green

A Parcel of Purple

A Reservoir of Red

A World of White

A Potpourri of Pink

Photo Credits

The artist/source credits for the photos in this book are listed in the order in which they appear:

Ryan M. Bolton/Shutterstock.com
Sergios/Shutterstock.com
troyka/Shutterstock.com
Patryk Kosmider/Shutterstock.com
Palo_ok/Shutterstock.com
Umkehrer/Shutterstock.com
Protasov AN/Shutterstock.com
E. O./Shutterstock.com
davemhuntphotography/Shutterstock.com
chungking/Shutterstock.com
Arina P Habich/Shutterstock.com
wannachat/Shutterstock.com
Kritchanut/Shutterstock.com
Alan Kraft/Shutterstock.com
www.sandatlas.org/Shutterstock.com
Nneirda/Shutterstock.com
Florin Stana/Shutterstock.com
dioch/Shutterstock.com
Doug Lemke/Shutterstock.com
Anton_Ivanov/Shutterstock.com
Inga Locmele/Shutterstock.com
Alexandra Giese/Shutterstock.com
Malgorzata Drewniak/Shutterstock.com

A Jellema/Shutterstock.com
Jung Hsuan/Shutterstock.com
grey color/Shutterstock.com
Vitaly Raduntsev/Shutterstock.com
odaodaodaod/Shutterstock.com
sanddebeautheil/Shutterstock.com
scubaluna/Shutterstock.com
Skynavin/Shutterstock.com
Butterfly Hunter/Shutterstock.com
grafnata/Shutterstock.com
cowardlion/Shutterstock.com
Bill Perry/Shutterstock.com
4n417/Shutterstock.com
Zanna Holstova/Shutterstock.com
SurangaSL/Shutterstock.com
patjo/Shutterstock.com
Rudra Narayan Mitra/Shutterstock.com
KoBoZaa/Shutterstock.com
Kristina Vackova/Shutterstock.com
Pal Teravagimov/Shutterstock.com
Ian Kennedy/Shutterstock.com
PerseoMedusa/Shutterstock.com
tea maeklong/Shutterstock.com

Made in United States
Orlando, FL
22 November 2022

24882220R00058